ANTI–CANCER FOODS

REDUCING YOUR RISK OF CANCER

BY
PASTOR ENGR EMEKA UNAEGBU
2024

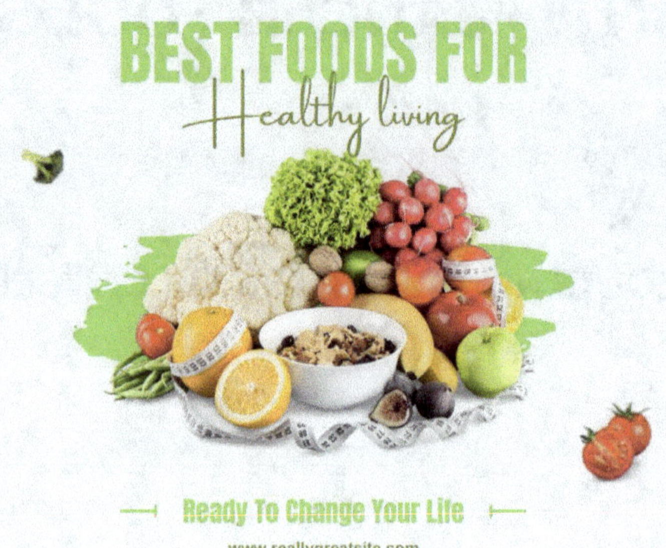

BEST FOODS FOR
Healthy living
Ready To Change Your Life
www.reallygreatsite.com

COPYRIGHT

@2024 Jumex Graphics, Apo, Abuja

Printed by Jumex Graphics, Chafuyi, Apo, Abuja FCT, Nigeria

Email: jumextng@gmail.com

Phone: +234 811 528 3445

DEDICATION

I greatly appreciate God for giving me this wonderful inspiration and ideas of writing to intervene and save humanity from the ravages of cancer.

ACKNOWLEDGEMENTS

My great thanks to my loving and caring wife – Mrs Uju Stella.

To my four wonderful kids Samuel, Angel, Goodluck and Vanessa for always inspiring me to do more.

For the staff and management of Jumex Transcontinental Limited for keeping hope alive, even in the most difficult times.

INTRODUCTION

In recent times, cancer has been one of the most deadly diseases ravaging humanity globally, it has been said, is the second most deadly killer of men and women globally after heart attack and heart related diseases.

To aggravate the situation, the causes of cancer is not well known but its manifestations are well known. Cancer incidences are wide and varied and could occur in any part of the body, could start from one part of the body and spread to others parts unnoticed.

Some cancer incidences are incurable but could be managed for the patient to live a normal life. The sickness has claimed the lives of important personalities globally including celebrities, men and women of God, politicians both high and mighty.

The good news is that there are few known ways of preventing cancer by consuming natural fruits and vegetables daily, exercising frequently but never extremely and quitting smoking which this book highlighted.

The book will embolden readers and practitioners never to panic about having cancer as they are in effect protected by the ravages of cancer if they put in practice what this book is saying.

A healthy diet can prevent tumors and cancers; thus, one should eat adequately and never more than one needs. One should limit their intake of calories and proteins. After smoking, being obese is the next leading reason which contributes to cancer rates.

It has been proven that though cancer incidences occur by genetic transfers from parents to offspring's, our lifestyle choices made over the course of years and decades control genetic expression and disease development and progression.

Organic foods are anti cancer healthy foods, but there should be no panic in consuming some types of foods as inorganic, hybrid, GMOs as these are insignificant to cancer incidences.

Practicing safe sex and staying away from toxic places, reduce the incidences of cancer. Exposure to toxic environments can lead to the development of malignancies like lung cancer and mesothelioma, anal cancer, throat cancer, cervical cancer and leukemia.

Two independent research bodies both provide firm evidence that the foods we consume directly impact our risk for developing cancer and can significantly lower cancer incidence.

An international study published on Nutrition explains that certain lifestyle factors, especially smoking and eating diets high in animal products, have strongest association with cancer rates. Investigators looked for 21 different forms of the disease from 157 different countries and statistically compared these rates with indices for risk modifying factors.

Junk food consumption is the second leading preventable cause of many types of cancer. The scientists explained, that smoking is the number one causes of cancers globally, while alcoholic beverage consumption is trailing as number three causes.

While smoking is the leading cause of cancer, the team found that animal products had the strongest correlation among certain cancers, including breast, kidney, ovarian, pancreatic, prostate, testicular and thyroid cancer.

A study group from Rutgers University has published the results of their work in the Journal of Clinical Endocrinology & Metabolism that demonstrates how adopting a diet rich in tomatoes may reduce the risk of developing breast cancer in at-risk groups of postmenopausal women. Research has shown that a recipe of tomatoes intake increases the level of adiponectin. Adiponectin is a hormone that plays a part in the regulation of fat and blood sugar levels and significantly lowers the risk for breast cancer incidence.

The study authors concluded, "Eating fruits and vegetables, which are rich in essential nutrients, vitamins, minerals and phytochemicals such as lycopene, conveys significant benefits. Based on this data, we believe regular consumption of at least the daily recommended servings of fruits and vegetables would promote breast cancer prevention in at-risk population". In addition to eliminating smoking as a fully accepted direct cause of cancer, adding a colorful variety of vegetables and fruits, especially lycopene-rich tomatoes, can impact gene expression to help prevent many forms of cancer.

Other fruits and vegetable that has anti cancer effects include broccoli, cabbage, cucumber, ginger, garlic and so many others.

This book will give some vital details in using fruits, vegetables, bodily exercise and positive thinking in living a life that is devoid of various cancers, thereby achieving good health and overall wellbeing for success in life, for health is wealth. A healthy man is a wealthy man.

Starting early to eat fruits and vegetables recipes will save you the agony of suffering the pains of various types of cancer in life for a stitch in time saves nine.

TABLE OF CONTENTS

CHAPTER ONE

WHAT IS CANCER?

Cancer is a disease that occurs when cells in the body grow uncontrollably and spread to other parts of the body. It is caused by changes to genes that control the way our cells function, especially how they grow and divide. Normally, human cells grow and multiply to form new cells as the body needs them. When cells grow old or become damaged, they die, and new cells take their place. Sometimes this orderly process breaks down, and abnormal or damaged cells grow and multiply when they shouldn't. These cells may form tumors, which are lumps of tissue. Tumors can be cancerous or not cancerous (benign). Cancerous tumors spread into, or invade, nearby tissues and can travel to distant places in the body to form new tumors (a process called metastasis). Cancerous tumors may also be called malignant tumors.

There are many different types of cancer, including breast cancer, lung cancer, and skin cancer. The symptoms of cancer depend on the type of cancer and the stage of the disease. Some common symptoms include fatigue, unexplained weight loss, pain, and skin changes. If you are concerned about cancer, it is important to talk to your doctor. They can help you understand your risk factors and recommend screening tests if necessary

WHAT ARE THE CAUSES OF CANCER?

Cancer is a group of diseases that occur when abnormal cells divide rapidly and can spread to other tissue and organs. The main cause of cancer is mutations, or changes to the DNA in your cells. Genetic mutations can be inherited or can occur after birth as a result of environmental factors, such as tobacco, alcohol, radiation, viruses, etc.

1.2 WHAT ARE DIFFERENT TYPES OF CANCER

There are many different types of cancer, each originating from different cells in the body. Some common types of cancer include:

1. Breast Cancer
2. Lung Cancer
3. Prostate Cancer
4. Colorectal Cancer
5. Skin Cancer (including melanoma and non-melanoma)
6. Leukemia

7. Lymphoma
8. Ovarian Cancer
9. Pancreatic Cancer
10. Liver Cancer
11. Bladder Cancer
12. Kidney Cancer
13. Brain Cancer
14. Thyroid Cancer
15. Cervical Cancer
16. Esophageal Cancer
17. Stomach Cancer
18. Testicular Cancer
19. Bone Cancer
20. Sarcoma (soft tissue and bone tumors)

It is important to note that there are many other types of cancer as well, and each type can have different subtypes or variations.

1.2 a. BREAST CANCER

Breast cancer is a type of cancer that develops in the cells of the breast. It is the most common cancer among women worldwide, but it can also affect men, although it is rare.

Breast cancer usually begins in the milk ducts (ductal carcinoma) or the lobules (lobular carcinoma) of the breast. It occurs when abnormal cells in the breast begin to grow and divide uncontrollably, forming a tumor. These cancerous cells can invade nearby tissues and spread to other parts of the body through the lymphatic system or bloodstream, a process known as metastasis.

Symptoms of breast cancer can vary, but common signs include a lump or thickening in the breast or underarm area, changes in breast size or shape, nipple changes or discharge, and skin changes on the breast. However, not all breast lumps are cancerous, and some breast cancers may not cause any symptoms at an early stage, which is why regular breast self-exams and mammograms are important for early detection.

Treatment for breast cancer may involve surgery, radiation therapy, chemotherapy, hormone therapy, targeted therapy, or a combination of these approaches. The choice of treatment depends on various factors, including the stage of cancer, the type of breast cancer, and the individual's overall health.

Early detection and advances in treatment have significantly improved the prognosis for breast cancer. Regular screenings, self-exams, and awareness of the risk factors can help in early detection and increase the chances of successful treatment.

b. LUNG CANCER

Lung cancer is a type of cancer that starts in the cells of the lungs. It is one of the most common types of cancer worldwide and is a leading cause of cancer-related deaths.

There are two main types of lung cancer: non-small cell lung cancer (NSCLC) and small cell lung cancer (SCLC). NSCLC is the most common type, accounting for about 85% of all lung cancers, while SCLC is less common but tends to grow and spread more rapidly.

Lung cancer typically develops when abnormal cells in the lungs begin to grow and divide uncontrollably, forming a tumor. These cancerous cells can then invade nearby tissues and spread to other parts of the body through the bloodstream or lymphatic system. Smoking is the leading cause of lung cancer, with exposure to secondhand smoke, radon, asbestos, and other environmental and occupational factors also contributing to the risk.

Symptoms of lung cancer can vary, but common signs include persistent cough, chest pain, shortness of breath, hoarseness, weight loss, fatigue, and recurrent respiratory infections. However, some people with lung cancer may not experience any symptoms until the disease has advanced.

Treatment options for lung cancer depend on the type and stage of cancer, as well as the individual's overall health. They may include surgery, radiation therapy, chemotherapy, targeted therapy, immunotherapy, or a combination of these approaches. Early detection through screenings, such as low-dose computed tomography (LDCT) scans, can improve the chances of successful treatment.

Prevention of lung cancer primarily involves avoiding tobacco smoke and reducing exposure to other known risk factors. Quitting smoking and maintaining a healthy lifestyle can significantly reduce the risk of developing lung cancer.

It is important to note that lung cancer can affect both smokers and non-smokers, and anyone experiencing symptoms or at risk should consult with a healthcare professional for proper evaluation and diagnosis.

c. PROSTATE CANCER

Prostate cancer is a type of cancer that occurs in the prostate gland, a small walnut-shaped gland located below the bladder in men. The prostate gland produces seminal fluid that nourishes and transports sperm.

Prostate cancer develops when the cells in the prostate gland grow and divide uncontrollably, forming a tumor. It is one of the most common types of cancer in men, but it typically grows slowly and may not cause noticeable symptoms in its early stages.

The exact cause of prostate cancer is unknown, but certain risk factors can increase the likelihood of developing the disease. These include age (prostate cancer is more common in older men), family history of prostate cancer, race (African-American men have a higher risk), and certain genetic mutations.

In its early stages, prostate cancer may not cause symptoms. However, as it progresses, symptoms may include difficulty urinating, weak urine flow, frequent urination (especially at night), blood in the urine or semen, erectile dysfunction, and pain or discomfort in the pelvic area.

Prostate cancer is typically diagnosed through a combination of a digital rectal examination (DRE), a blood test called prostate-specific antigen (PSA) test, and possibly a prostate biopsy to confirm the presence of cancer cells.

Treatment options for prostate cancer depend on various factors, including the stage and aggressiveness of the cancer, the age and overall health of the individual, and personal preferences. Treatment options may include active surveillance (monitoring the cancer without immediate treatment), surgery, radiation therapy, hormone therapy, chemotherapy, or immunotherapy.

Regular screenings and early detection are crucial for the successful treatment of prostate cancer. Men should discuss the potential benefits and risks of prostate cancer screening with their healthcare providers to make informed decisions about when to begin screening and how often to undergo testing.

It's important to note that each individual's experience with prostate cancer can vary, and consulting with a healthcare professional is essential for proper evaluation, diagnosis, and treatment planning.

d. LEUKEMIA OR BLOOD CANCER

Leukemia, also known as blood cancer, is a type of cancer that affects the bone marrow and blood. It occurs when there is an abnormal production of white blood cells, which are responsible for fighting infection and maintaining the body's immune system.

Leukemia can be classified into different types based on the specific type of white blood cell affected and the rate of disease progression. The main types of leukemia include:

1. Acute Lymphoblastic Leukemia (ALL): This type of leukemia primarily affects lymphoid cells, which are a type of white blood cell. It is more common in children, but it can also occur in adults.

2. Acute Myeloid Leukemia (AML): AML affects myeloid cells, which are another type of white blood cell. It can occur in both children and adults.

3. Chronic Lymphocytic Leukemia (CLL): CLL is characterized by the slow accumulation of abnormal lymphocytes, a type of white blood cell. It is more common in older adults.

4. Chronic Myeloid Leukemia (CML): CML affects myeloid cells and is often associated with the presence of a specific genetic abnormality known as the Philadelphia chromosome. It can occur in all age groups, but it is more common in older adults.

Leukemia can cause a range of symptoms, including fatigue, weakness, frequent infections, easy bleeding or bruising, weight loss, swollen lymph nodes, and bone or joint pain. However, some people with leukemia may not experience any symptoms initially, and the disease may be detected through routine blood tests.

The exact cause of leukemia is often unknown, but certain risk factors can increase the likelihood of developing the disease. These include exposure to high levels of radiation or certain chemicals, certain genetic conditions, previous chemotherapy or radiation therapy, and a family history of leukemia.

Treatment for leukemia depends on the specific type, stage, and individual factors. Common treatment options include chemotherapy, targeted therapy, radiation therapy, stem cell transplantation, and immunotherapy. The treatment plan is tailored to each individual's needs and may involve a combination of these approaches.

Advancements in treatment have significantly improved the prognosis for many people with leukemia. However, the outlook can vary depending on factors such as the type and stage of leukemia, age, overall health, and response to treatment.

If you suspect any symptoms or have concerns about leukemia, it is important to consult with a healthcare professional for proper evaluation, diagnosis, and treatment recommendations.

e. LIVER CANCER

Liver cancer, also known as hepatocellular carcinoma (HCC), is a type of cancer that originates in the cells of the liver. It is the sixth most common cancer worldwide and often occurs in individuals with underlying liver diseases, such as cirrhosis or chronic hepatitis B or C infections.

The liver plays a vital role in various bodily functions, including filtering toxins from the blood, producing bile for digestion, and storing nutrients. Liver cancer typically develops when normal liver cells undergo genetic mutations, leading to uncontrolled growth and the formation of tumors.

THERE ARE TWO PRIMARY TYPES OF LIVER CANCER:

1. PRIMARY LIVER CANCER:

This refers to cancers that originate in the liver itself. Hepatocellular carcinoma (HCC) is the most common type of primary liver cancer and accounts for the majority of cases.

ANTI-CANCER FOODS | By Pst. Engr. Emeka Unaegbu

2. **SECONDARY LIVER CANCER:**
   Also known as metastatic liver cancer, this occurs when cancer cells from other parts of the body spread to the liver. The liver is a common site for metastasis due to its abundant blood supply.

Liver cancer may not cause noticeable symptoms in its early stages. As the disease progresses, symptoms may include abdominal pain or swelling, unexplained weight loss, loss of appetite, fatigue, yellowing of the skin or eyes (jaundice), and changes in bowel movements.

Several risk factors can increase the likelihood of developing liver cancer. These include chronic hepatitis B or C infections, excessive alcohol consumption, obesity, diabetes, exposure to certain chemicals or toxins, and certain genetic conditions.

Diagnosing liver cancer typically involves imaging tests such as ultrasound, CT scan, or MRI, as well as blood tests to assess liver function and tumor markers. A liver biopsy may be performed to confirm the diagnosis.

Treatment options for liver cancer depend on various factors, including the stage of cancer, the individual's overall health, and the extent of liver damage. Treatment may involve surgery to remove the tumor, liver transplantation, radiation therapy, targeted therapy, chemotherapy, or a combination of these approaches.

Prevention of liver cancer involves reducing risk factors such as practicing safe sex, getting vaccinated against hepatitis B, limiting alcohol consumption, maintaining a healthy weight, and avoiding exposure to toxins and chemicals.

Early detection and timely treatment are crucial for improving the prognosis of liver cancer. Regular check-ups, screenings, and seeking medical attention for any concerning symptoms are essential. Consulting with a healthcare professional can provide personalized guidance and recommendations based on individual circumstances.

f. TESTICULAR CANCER

Testicular cancer is a type of cancer that develops in the testicles, which are the male reproductive organs responsible for producing sperm and testosterone. It is relatively rare compared to other types of cancer but is the most common cancer in males aged 15 to 35.

Testicular cancer typically begins in the germ cells, which are the cells that produce immature sperm. There are two main types of testicular cancer:

1. **Seminoma:** This type of testicular cancer usually grows slowly and is more responsive to radiation therapy. It tends to occur in men in their 30s and 40s.

2. **Non-seminoma:** Non-seminoma testicular cancer is more aggressive and tends to grow and spread more quickly. It often occurs in younger men, typically in their late teens or early 20s.

The exact cause of testicular cancer is unknown, but certain risk factors have been identified. These include undescended testicles (cryptorchidism), family history of testicular cancer, previous history of testicular cancer, and certain genetic conditions.

Common signs and symptoms of testicular cancer may include a painless lump or swelling in the testicle, a feeling of heaviness or discomfort in the scrotum, pain or discomfort in the testicle or scrotum, changes in testicle size or shape, and a dull ache in the lower abdomen or groin.

ANTI-CANCER FOODS | By Pst. Engr. Emeka Unaegbu

Early detection and diagnosis of testicular cancer are crucial for successful treatment. Self-examination of the testicles can help men identify any changes or abnormalities. If a lump or other concerning symptoms are present, it is important to consult a healthcare professional for further evaluation.

Treatment options for testicular cancer depend on the type and stage of cancer, as well as individual factors. Common treatments include surgery to remove the affected testicle (called radical inguinal orchiectomy), radiation therapy, chemotherapy, and sometimes surveillance (active monitoring) for certain low-risk cases.

The prognosis for testicular cancer is generally favorable, with high cure rates, especially for early-stage cancers. Regular follow-up care and monitoring are important to detect any potential recurrences or complications.

It is important for men to be aware of their testicular health, perform regular self-examinations, and seek medical attention if any changes or concerns arise. Consulting with a healthcare professional can provide personalized guidance and recommendations based on individual circumstances.

g. STOMACH CANCER

Stomach cancer, also known as gastric cancer, is a type of cancer that develops in the cells lining the stomach. It is a relatively common cancer worldwide, although its incidence has been decreasing in many countries.

Stomach cancer typically begins in the innermost layer of the stomach and can spread to other parts of the organ or nearby lymph nodes. There are several types of stomach cancer, including adenocarcinoma (the most common type), lymphoma, gastrointestinal stromal tumor (GIST), and carcinoid tumor.

The exact cause of stomach cancer is not fully understood, but certain risk factors have been identified. These include infection with Helicobacter pylori bacteria, a diet high in smoked, salted, or pickled foods, a family history of stomach cancer, smoking, obesity, and certain genetic conditions.

Stomach cancer often does not cause noticeable symptoms in its early stages. As the disease progresses, symptoms may include persistent indigestion, heartburn, abdominal pain or discomfort, unintentional weight loss, loss of appetite, nausea, vomiting (sometimes with blood), difficulty swallowing, and black, tarry stools.

Diagnosing stomach cancer typically involves a combination of medical history evaluation, physical examination, imaging tests (such as CT scan or endoscopy), and a biopsy to examine tissue samples for cancer cells.

Treatment options for stomach cancer depend on various factors, including the stage of cancer, the location and size of the tumor, and the overall health of the individual. Treatment may involve surgery to remove part or all of the stomach, chemotherapy, radiation therapy, targeted therapy, or a combination of these approaches.

Prevention of stomach cancer involves reducing risk factors such as treating Helicobacter pylori infection, adopting a healthy diet rich in fruits and vegetables, avoiding excessive consumption of processed or smoked foods, quitting smoking, maintaining a healthy weight, and seeking early treatment for gastrointestinal conditions such as gastritis or ulcers.

The prognosis for stomach cancer varies depending on the stage at diagnosis and other individual factors. Early detection and timely treatment can improve outcomes. Regular check-ups, screenings, and seeking medical attention for any concerning symptoms are important.

If you have any concerns or suspect any symptoms related to stomach cancer, it is important to consult with a healthcare professional for proper evaluation, diagnosis, and treatment recommendations.

h. BONE CANCER

Bone cancer refers to a type of cancer that originates in the bones. It can occur in any bone in the body, but most commonly affects the long bones of the arms and legs. There are several types of bone cancer, including primary bone cancer and secondary bone cancer.

Primary bone cancer starts in the bone itself and can be further classified into different types, such as osteosarcoma, Ewing sarcoma, and chondrosarcoma. Osteosarcoma is the most common type and often affects children and young adults, while chondrosarcoma typically occurs in older adults. Ewing sarcoma is more common in children and teenagers.

Secondary bone cancer, also known as metastatic bone cancer, occurs when cancer cells from another part of the body spread to the bones. Common types of cancer that can metastasize to the bones include breast, lung, prostate, and kidney cancer.

The exact cause of primary bone cancer is often unknown, but certain risk factors have been identified. These include previous radiation therapy, certain genetic conditions like Li-Fraumeni syndrome and hereditary retinoblastoma, and certain inherited bone diseases.

The symptoms of bone cancer can vary depending on the location and stage of the cancer. Common symptoms may include bone pain (which may worsen at night or with activity), swelling or a lump in the affected area, fractures or bone weakening, fatigue, weight loss, and anemia.

Diagnosing bone cancer typically involves a combination of medical history evaluation, physical examination, imaging tests (such as X-rays, CT scans, MRI, or bone scans), and a biopsy to examine tissue samples for cancer cells.

Treatment options for bone cancer depend on various factors, including the type, stage, and location of the cancer, as well as the individual's overall health. Treatment may involve surgery to remove the tumor, chemotherapy, radiation therapy, targeted therapy, or a combination of these approaches.

The prognosis for bone cancer varies depending on the type, stage, and other individual factors. Early detection and treatment can improve outcomes. Regular check-ups, screenings, and seeking medical attention for any concerning symptoms are important.

If you have any concerns or suspect any symptoms related to bone cancer, it is important to consult with a healthcare professional for proper evaluation, diagnosis, and treatment recommendations.

1.3 WHAT ARE THE IMPORTANCE OF DIET IN CANCER PREVENTION

Diet plays a crucial role in cancer prevention. While it is not a guarantee against developing cancer, maintaining a healthy diet can significantly reduce the risk of certain types of cancer. Here are some key reasons why diet is important in cancer prevention:

1. **NUTRIENT-RICH FOODS**:
   A balanced and nutrient-rich diet provides the body with essential vitamins, minerals, antioxidants, and other beneficial compounds that support overall health and strengthen the immune system. This can help the body in fighting against the development and progression of cancer cells.

2. **WEIGHT MANAGEMENT**:

Obesity and excess body weight have been linked to an increased risk of several types of cancer, including breast, colorectal, kidney, and pancreatic cancer. A healthy diet that is low in calorie-dense foods and high in fruits, vegetables, whole grains, and lean proteins can help maintain a healthy weight and reduce the risk of obesity-related cancers.

3. **ANTIOXIDANTS AND PHYTOCHEMICALS**:

Fruits, vegetables, whole grains, and legumes are rich in antioxidants and phytochemicals, which are compounds that have been shown to have cancer-fighting properties. These compounds help protect cells from damage caused by free radicals and inflammation, which can contribute to cancer development.

4. **FIBER INTAKE:**

A diet high in fiber, which is found in fruits, vegetables, whole grains, and legumes, has been associated with a reduced risk of colorectal cancer. Fiber helps promote regular bowel movements, which can help eliminate potential carcinogens from the body and prevent the formation of cancerous cells.

5. **REDUCED INTAKE OF PROCESSED AND RED MEATS**:

Consumption of processed meats, such as bacon, sausages, and deli meats, as well as high consumption of red meats, has been linked to an increased risk of colorectal and other types of cancer. Limiting the intake of these foods and opting for lean protein sources like poultry, fish, and plant-based proteins can help reduce the risk.

6. **DECREASED INTAKE OF SUGARY AND PROCESSED FOODS:**

A diet high in sugary and processed foods has been associated with an increased risk of obesity, type 2 diabetes, and certain types of cancer. Limiting the consumption of sugary drinks, processed snacks, and desserts can contribute to a healthier diet and lower cancer risk.

It is important to note that while diet is an important aspect of cancer prevention, it should be considered as part of an overall healthy lifestyle. Regular physical activity, avoiding tobacco and excessive alcohol consumption, and maintaining a healthy weight are also crucial factors in reducing the risk of cancer.

CHAPTER TWO

UNDERSTANDING THE ROLE OF MACRO NUTRIENTS IN CANCER PREVENTION

2.0 WHAT ARE MACRO NUTRIENTS

Macronutrients are the essential nutrients that our bodies need in large quantities to function properly. They include carbohydrates, proteins, and fats. Carbohydrates are the body's main source of energy, proteins are essential for growth and repair of tissues, and fats provide energy, insulation, and support various bodily functions. It is important to have a balanced intake of macronutrients to maintain good health.

2.1 CARBOHYDRATES AND CANCER PREVENTION

Carbohydrates play several important roles in cancer prevention:

a. **DIETARY FIBER:**
Carbohydrates are a major source of dietary fiber, which is essential for maintaining a healthy digestive system. High-fiber diets have been linked to a

reduced risk of various types of cancer, including colorectal cancer. Fiber helps to promote regular bowel movements, prevent constipation, and eliminate toxins from the body.

b. **ANTIOXIDANTS:**
Many carbohydrate-rich foods, such as fruits, vegetables, and whole grains, are rich in antioxidants. Antioxidants help to neutralize harmful free radicals in the body, which can cause damage to cells and DNA, leading to cancer development. By consuming a diet high in carbohydrates that are rich in antioxidants, you can help protect your cells from oxidative stress and reduce the risk of cancer.

c. **ENERGY SOURCE:**
Carbohydrates are the body's primary source of energy. By consuming a balanced diet that includes complex carbohydrates, such as whole grains, legumes, and starchy vegetables, you can maintain a healthy weight and reduce the risk of obesity. Obesity is a known risk factor for several types of cancer, including breast, colorectal, and pancreatic cancer.

d. **GLYCEMIC INDEX:**
Carbohydrates have different glycemic indexes, which measure how quickly they raise blood sugar

levels. High-glycemic index carbohydrates, such as refined sugars and processed foods, can cause rapid spikes in blood sugar levels. These spikes can lead to chronic inflammation and insulin resistance, which are risk factors for cancer. Choosing low-glycemic index carbohydrates, such as whole grains, fruits, and vegetables, can help regulate blood sugar levels and reduce the risk of cancer.

It's important to note that while carbohydrates can play a role in cancer prevention, it's also essential to maintain a balanced diet that includes other nutrients, such as proteins, healthy fats, vitamins, and minerals. Additionally, it's always recommended to consult with a healthcare professional or registered dietitian for personalized dietary advice.

2.2 PROTEINS AND CANCER PREVENTION

Proteins play several important roles in cancer prevention:

a. **CELL GROWTH AND REPAIR:**
   Proteins are essential for the growth, repair, and maintenance of cells in the body. They are involved in the synthesis and regulation of DNA, RNA, and various enzymes. By consuming an adequate amount of protein, you can support healthy cell

growth and repair damaged cells, which can help prevent the development of cancer.

b. **IMMUNE FUNCTION:**
Proteins are crucial for a strong immune system. They help produce antibodies, which are proteins that recognize and neutralize foreign substances, such as viruses and bacteria. A robust immune system is essential for identifying and eliminating cancer cells before they can develop into tumors. Consuming sufficient protein can support optimal immune function and enhance the body's ability to fight off cancer.

c. **ANTIOXIDANT PRODUCTION:**
Some proteins, such as glutathione, act as antioxidants in the body. Antioxidants help neutralize harmful free radicals, which can cause DNA damage and contribute to cancer development. By consuming protein-rich foods, you can support the production of antioxidants and enhance the body's defense against oxidative stress.

d. **MUSCLE MAINTENANCE:**
Adequate protein intake is crucial for maintaining muscle mass and strength. Regular physical activity, including strength training, has been shown to reduce the risk of certain cancers, such as colon,

breast, and endometrial cancer. Protein plays a vital role in muscle repair and growth, which can help support an active lifestyle and reduce the risk of cancer.

It's important to note that while proteins are essential for cancer prevention, it's also crucial to consume a balanced diet that includes carbohydrates, healthy fats, vitamins, and minerals. Additionally, individual protein needs may vary depending on factors such as age, sex, activity level, and overall health. Consulting with a healthcare professional or registered dietitian can provide personalized guidance on protein intake for cancer prevention.

2.3 FATS AND OILS IN CANCER PREVENTION

Fats and oils play several important roles in cancer prevention:

1. **ESSENTIAL FATTY ACIDS:**
   Fats are a primary source of essential fatty acids, such as omega-3 and omega-6 fatty acids. These fatty acids are crucial for maintaining healthy cell membranes, regulating inflammation, and supporting immune function. By consuming a balanced diet that includes sources of healthy fats, such as fatty fish, nuts, seeds, and avocados, you

can help reduce chronic inflammation and support overall health, which can contribute to cancer prevention.

2. **FAT-SOLUBLE VITAMINS:**
Some vitamins, such as vitamins A, D, E, and K, are fat-soluble, meaning they require fat for absorption and utilization in the body. These vitamins have antioxidant properties and play important roles in cell growth, immune function, and DNA repair. By consuming fats and oils in moderation, you can enhance the absorption of these vitamins and support their cancer-preventive effects.

3. **ENERGY SOURCE:**
Fats are a concentrated source of energy, providing more than twice the calories per gram compared to carbohydrates and proteins. By consuming healthy fats in moderation, you can maintain a healthy weight and reduce the risk of obesity, which is a known risk factor for several types of cancer.

4. **PHYTOCHEMICALS:**
Some fats and oils, such as those derived from plant sources like olives, avocados, and nuts, contain phytochemicals. These natural compounds have been shown to have anti-inflammatory and

antioxidant properties, which can help protect against DNA damage and reduce the risk of cancer.

It's important to note that not all fats and oils are created equal. Consuming excessive amounts of unhealthy fats, such as Tran's fats and saturated fats found in processed foods and fatty meats, can increase the risk of cancer and other chronic diseases. It's recommended to focus on consuming healthy fats from sources like nuts, seeds, avocados, olive oil, and fatty fish, while limiting the intake of unhealthy fats.

As always, it's advisable to consult with a healthcare professional or registered dietitian for personalized dietary advice, especially if you have specific health concerns or conditions.

CHAPTER THREE

INCORPORATING ANTI-OXIDANT RICH FOODS IN YOUR DIET

Antioxidant-rich foods are those that contain high levels of compounds that can help neutralize harmful free radicals in the body. Here are some examples of antioxidant-rich foods:

1. **BERRIES:**
   Blueberries, strawberries, raspberries, and blackberries are all excellent sources of antioxidants, particularly anthocyanins. These compounds give berries their vibrant colors and have been linked to various health benefits, including reducing inflammation and protecting against cancer.

2. **DARK CHOCOLATE:**
   Dark chocolate, particularly those with a high cocoa content (70% or more), is rich in antioxidants called flavonoids. These antioxidants have been shown to have anti-inflammatory and heart-protective effects. However, it's important to consume dark chocolate in moderation due to its calorie and sugar content.

3. **LEAFY GREEN VEGETABLES:**
Spinach, kale, Swiss chard, and other leafy greens are packed with antioxidants such as vitamin C, vitamin E, and beta-carotene. These antioxidants help protect cells from damage and reduce the risk of chronic diseases, including cancer and heart disease.

4. **NUTS AND SEEDS**:
Almonds, walnuts, flaxseeds, and chia seeds are all good sources of antioxidants, healthy fats, and fiber. They provide a range of antioxidants, including vitamin E, selenium, and various phytochemicals, which help reduce inflammation and oxidative stress in the body.

5. **COLORFUL FRUITS:**
Fruits like oranges, grapes, pomegranates, and kiwis are rich in antioxidants, including vitamin C and various flavonoids. These antioxidants help boost the immune system, protect against cell damage, and reduce the risk of chronic diseases.

6. **GREEN TEA**:
Green tea contains polyphenols, particularly catechins, which are potent antioxidants. Regular consumption of green tea has been associated with

a reduced risk of various cancers, improved heart health, and enhanced brain function.

7. **SPICES AND HERBS:**
   Many spices and herbs are known for their antioxidant properties. Examples include turmeric, cinnamon, ginger, cloves, oregano, and rosemary. These can be incorporated into meals and beverages to add flavor and increase antioxidant intake.

It's important to note that a balanced and varied diet, rich in whole foods, is the best way to obtain a wide range of antioxidants and other beneficial nutrients. Aim to include a variety of antioxidant-rich foods in your diet to maximize their health benefits.

3.1 IMPORTANCE OF ANTIOXIDANTS IN CANCER PREVENTION

Antioxidants play a crucial role in cancer prevention due to their ability to neutralize harmful free radicals in the body. Here are some important reasons why antioxidants are beneficial in preventing cancer:

1. **NEUTRALIZING FREE RADICALS:**
   Free radicals are unstable molecules that can damage DNA, proteins, and other cellular

structures, leading to the development of cancer. Antioxidants help neutralize these free radicals, preventing them from causing oxidative stress and reducing the risk of cancer.

2. **DNA PROTECTION:**
Antioxidants can protect the integrity of DNA, which is essential for preventing mutations that can lead to the development of cancer cells. By preventing DNA damage, antioxidants help maintain the normal functioning of cells and reduce the risk of cancerous growth.

3. **ANTI-INFLAMMATORY EFFECTS:**
Chronic inflammation is closely linked to the development of cancer. Antioxidants have anti-inflammatory properties, helping to reduce inflammation in the body. By reducing inflammation, antioxidants help create an environment less conducive to cancer growth.

4. **IMMUNE SYSTEM SUPPORT:**
Antioxidants can strengthen the immune system, which plays a vital role in identifying and eliminating cancer cells. A strong immune system is better equipped to detect and destroy abnormal cells, reducing the risk of cancer development.

5. **PROTECTION AGAINST CARCINOGENS:**
Antioxidants can help protect against exposure to carcinogens, which are substances that have the potential to cause cancer. By neutralizing carcinogens and preventing them from damaging cells, antioxidants contribute to cancer prevention.

6. **PROMOTION OF HEALTHY CELL GROWTH:**
Antioxidants support healthy cell growth and division, which is essential for maintaining the normal functioning of tissues and organs. By promoting healthy cell growth, antioxidants help prevent the uncontrolled growth of cancer cells.

7. **ENHANCEMENT OF CHEMOTHERAPY EFFECTIVENESS:**
Some studies suggest that antioxidants, when used in conjunction with chemotherapy, can enhance the effectiveness of the treatment. They may help protect healthy cells from damage caused by chemotherapy while sensitizing cancer cells to the treatment.

It is important to note that while antioxidants have potential benefits in cancer prevention, they should be obtained from a balanced diet rather than through supplements. A varied diet rich in fruits, vegetables, whole grains, and legumes can provide a wide range of antioxidants along with other beneficial nutrients.

3.2 TOP ANTIOXIDANTS-RICH FOODS TO INCLUDE IN YOUR DIETS

Including antioxidant-rich foods in your diet can provide numerous health benefits. Here are some examples of foods that are high in antioxidants:

1. **BERRIES:**
   Blueberries, strawberries, raspberries, and blackberries are all excellent sources of antioxidants such as anthocyanins and vitamin C.

2. **DARK CHOCOLATE:**
   Dark chocolate with a high cocoa content contains flavonoids, which act as antioxidants. Look for chocolate with at least 70% cocoa content for maximum benefits.

3. **GREEN LEAFY VEGETABLES**:
   Spinach, kale, and Swiss chard are rich in antioxidants such as vitamin C, vitamin E, and beta-carotene.

4. **NUTS AND SEEDS:**
Almonds, walnuts, flaxseeds, and chia seeds are packed with antioxidants like vitamin E, selenium, and polyphenols.

5. **COLORFUL FRUITS:**
Citrus fruits like oranges and grapefruits, as well as other fruits like kiwi, papaya, and mango, are rich in antioxidants such as vitamin C and beta-carotene.

6. **CRUCIFEROUS VEGETABLES:**
Broccoli, cauliflower, Brussels sprouts, and cabbage are high in antioxidants like sulforaphane and indole-3-carbinol.

7. **SPICES:**
Turmeric, cinnamon, ginger, and cloves are spices that contain potent antioxidants like curcumin and gingerol.

8. **BEANS AND LEGUMES:**
Kidney beans, black beans, lentils, and chickpeas are excellent sources of antioxidants like flavonoids and anthocyanins.

9. **WHOLE GRAINS:**
Foods like brown rice, quinoa, and oats contain antioxidants such as selenium and phenolic acids.

 ANTI-CANCER FOODS | By Pst. Engr. Emeka Unaegbu

10. **GREEN TEA:**
Green tea is rich in catechins, which are powerful antioxidants that can help protect against various diseases.

Remember, it's best to obtain antioxidants through a varied and balanced diet rather than relying on supplements. Aim to include a variety of these antioxidant-rich foods in your daily meals to maximize their benefits.

3.3 RECIPES AND MEAL IDEAS TO BOOST ANTIOXIDANT INTAKE

Here are some recipe and meal ideas to help boost your antioxidant intake:

a. **BERRY SMOOTHIE BOWL:**
- Blend a mix of berries (such as blueberries, strawberries, and raspberries) with a banana and your choice of liquid (milk, yogurt, or plant-based milk).
- Pour the smoothie into a bowl and top it with sliced fruits, nuts, seeds, and a sprinkle of granola for added crunch.

b. COLORFUL SALAD:

- Combine a variety of antioxidant-rich vegetables like spinach, kale, bell peppers, cherry tomatoes, and grated carrots.
- Add some protein like grilled chicken, salmon, or tofu.
- Drizzle with a homemade dressing made with olive oil, lemon juice, and herbs.

c. QUINOA AND ROASTED VEGETABLE BOWL:

- Cook quinoa according to package instructions.
- Roast a mix of antioxidant-rich vegetables like broccoli, cauliflower, sweet potatoes, and red onions with olive oil, salt, and pepper.
- Serve the roasted vegetables over a bed of quinoa and top with a sprinkle of feta cheese or toasted nuts.

d. GREEN TEA INFUSED SALMON:

- Marinate salmon fillets in a mixture of green tea, soy sauce, garlic, and ginger for at least 30 minutes.
- Grill or bake the salmon until cooked through.
- Serve with a side of steamed vegetables and brown rice.

e. **DARK CHOCOLATE AND BERRY PARFAIT:**

- Layer Greek yogurt, mixed berries, and dark chocolate chunks in a glass or jar.
- Repeat the layers until the glass is filled.
- Top with a dollop of Greek yogurt and a sprinkle of chopped nuts.

f. **TURMERIC ROASTED CAULIFLOWER:**

- Toss cauliflower florets with olive oil, turmeric, cumin, salt, and pepper.
- Roast in the oven until golden and tender.
- Serve as a side dish or add to salads or grain bowls.

Remember, these are just a few ideas, and you can get creative by incorporating antioxidant-rich ingredients into various dishes. Experiment with different fruits, vegetables, herbs, and spices to maximize your antioxidant intake while enjoying delicious and nutritious meals.

CHAPTER FOUR

THE POWER OF PHYTOCHEMICALS IN CANCER PREVENTION

4.1 WHAT ARE PHYTOCHEMICALS AND HOW DO THEY WORK

Phytochemicals, also known as phytonutrients, are natural compounds found in plants. They are responsible for the vibrant colors, flavors, and aromas of fruits, vegetables, grains, legumes, herbs, and spices. Phytochemicals are not considered essential nutrients like vitamins and minerals, but they have been found to have numerous health benefits.

Phytochemicals work in various ways to promote health and protect against diseases. Here are some mechanisms by which phytochemicals exert their effects:

a. **ANTIOXIDANT ACTIVITY:**
   Many phytochemicals act as antioxidants, which means they can neutralize harmful free radicals in the body. Free radicals are unstable molecules that can damage cells and contribute to chronic diseases like cancer, heart disease, and aging. By neutralizing free radicals, phytochemicals help

reduce oxidative stress and protect cells from damage.

b. **ANTI-INFLAMMATORY EFFECTS**:
Chronic inflammation is associated with various diseases, including cancer, diabetes, and cardiovascular disease. Some phytochemicals have anti-inflammatory properties, helping to reduce inflammation in the body. By reducing inflammation, these compounds can help prevent and manage chronic diseases.

c. **DETOXIFICATION SUPPORT:**
Certain phytochemicals can enhance the body's natural detoxification processes. They can stimulate enzymes involved in detoxification and elimination of harmful substances, such as carcinogens and environmental toxins.

d. **HORMONAL MODULATION**:
Some phytochemicals can interact with hormone receptors and modulate hormone production and activity. For example, isoflavones found in soybeans can mimic or block estrogen in the body, which may have protective effects against hormone-related cancers.

e. **IMMUNE SYSTEM SUPPORT**:
Phytochemicals can help support a healthy immune system by enhancing immune cell function and promoting the production of antibodies. This can help the body defend against infections and diseases.

f. **ANTI-CANCER PROPERTIES:**
Many phytochemicals have been studied for their potential anti-cancer effects. They can inhibit the growth of cancer cells, induce cell death (apoptosis), and prevent the formation of new blood vessels that supply nutrients to tumors (angiogenesis).

It's important to note that the specific mechanisms of action and health benefits vary for different phytochemicals. Therefore, consuming a diverse range of plant-based foods is key to obtaining a wide variety of phytochemicals and maximizing their potential health benefits.

4.2 PHYTOCHEMICAL-RICH FOODS FOR CANCER PREVENTION

Including phytochemical-rich foods in your diet can contribute to cancer prevention. Here are some examples of foods that are particularly rich in phytochemicals:

1. **CRUCIFEROUS VEGETABLES**:
    Broccoli, cauliflower, Brussels sprouts, kale, and cabbage are rich in phytochemicals such as glucosinolates, which have been associated with a reduced risk of various cancers, including lung, colorectal, and breast cancer.

2. **BERRIES:**
    Blueberries, strawberries, raspberries, and blackberries are packed with phytochemicals like anthocyanins, which have antioxidant and anti-inflammatory properties that may help protect against cancer.

3. **TOMATOES:**
    Tomatoes contain the phytochemical lycopene, which has been linked to a lower risk of certain cancers, including prostate, lung, and stomach cancer. Cooking tomatoes can enhance the absorption of lycopene.

4. **GREEN TEA:**
    Green tea is rich in catechins, a type of phytochemical that has been studied for its potential anti-cancer properties. Regular consumption of

green tea has been associated with a reduced risk of several cancers, including breast, prostate, and colorectal cancer.

5. **GARLIC AND ONIONS:**

Garlic and onions contain organosulfur compounds, such as allicin, which have been shown to have anti-cancer effects. These compounds may help inhibit the growth of cancer cells and reduce the risk of stomach, colorectal, and prostate cancer.

6. **TURMERIC:**

Turmeric contains the phytochemical curcumin, which has potent anti-inflammatory and antioxidant properties. Curcumin has been studied for its potential in preventing and treating various types of cancer, including colorectal, breast, and pancreatic cancer.

7. **CITRUS FRUITS:**

Citrus fruits like oranges, lemons, and grapefruits are rich in phytochemicals such as flavonoids and limonoids, which have been associated with a reduced risk of certain cancers, including esophageal, stomach, and pancreatic cancer.

8. **LEGUMES:**
Legumes like beans, lentils, and chickpeas are excellent sources of phytochemicals such as flavonoids and lignans, which have been linked to a lower risk of breast, colorectal, and prostate cancer.

9. **DARK LEAFY GREENS**:
Spinach, kale, Swiss chard, and other dark leafy greens are rich in phytochemicals like carotenoids, flavonoids, and chlorophyll, which have been associated with a reduced risk of various cancers, including lung, stomach, and colorectal cancer.

10. **WHOLE GRAINS:**
Whole grains like brown rice, quinoa, oats, and whole wheat contain phytochemicals such as lignans and phenolic acids, which have been linked to a lower risk of several cancers, including breast, colorectal, and pancreatic cancer.

Incorporating a variety of these phytochemical-rich foods into your diet can provide a wide range of cancer-fighting compounds. Remember to consume them as part of a balanced and varied diet for maximum benefits.

4.3 TIPS OF INCORPORATING PHOTOCHEMICALS INTO YOUR DIETS

Here are some tips for incorporating phytochemicals into your diet:

1. **EAT A VARIETY OF COLORFUL FRUITS AND VEGETABLES**:
   Phytochemicals are responsible for the vibrant colors in fruits and vegetables, so aim to include a wide range of colors in your diet. Include red, orange, yellow, green, blue, and purple produce to ensure you're getting a diverse array of phytochemicals.

2. **Choose whole foods over supplements**: While supplements can be beneficial in certain cases, it's generally best to obtain phytochemicals from whole foods. Whole foods provide a combination of phytochemicals, fiber, vitamins, and minerals that work synergistically for optimal health.

3. **INCORPORATE HERBS AND SPICES:**
   Herbs and spices are excellent sources of phytochemicals. Add flavor and phytochemical-rich ingredients like turmeric, ginger, garlic, cinnamon, oregano, and basil to your dishes.

4. **INCLUDE LEGUMES IN YOUR MEALS:**
Legumes, such as beans, lentils, and chickpeas, are rich in phytochemicals. They are also high in fiber and protein, making them a nutritious addition to your diet. Try adding them to soups, salads, or as a side dish.

5. **SNACK ON NUTS AND SEEDS:**
Nuts and seeds are packed with phytochemicals, healthy fats, and other nutrients. Enjoy a handful of almonds, walnuts, sunflower seeds, or flaxseeds as a snack or sprinkle them over salads, yogurt, or oatmeal.

6. **OPT FOR WHOLE GRAINS:**
Whole grains like brown rice, quinoa, oats, and whole wheat contain phytochemicals that are beneficial for your health. Choose whole grain options over refined grains to maximize your phytochemical intake.

7. **INCLUDE CRUCIFEROUS VEGETABLES:**
Cruciferous vegetables like broccoli, cauliflower, kale, and Brussels sprouts are rich in phytochemicals known as glucosinolates. These compounds have been associated with various health benefits, including cancer prevention.

ANTI-CANCER FOODS | By Pst. Engr. Emeka Unaegbu

Incorporate them into stir-fries, salads, or roasted vegetable dishes.

8. **MAKE SMOOTHIES OR JUICES**:
   Smoothies and juices can be a great way to incorporate a variety of fruits and vegetables into your diet. Blend or juice a combination of colorful produce to create a nutrient-rich beverage that is high in phytochemicals.

Remember, it's important to consult with a healthcare professional or registered dietitian for personalized advice and guidance on incorporating phytochemicals into your diet.

CHAPTER FIVE

THE ROLE OF FIBER IN CANCER PREVENTION

5.1 UNDERSTANDING THE BENEFITS OF DIETARY FIBER

Dietary fiber has numerous benefits for our health. Here are some key benefits of including an adequate amount of dietary fiber in your diet:

1. **Improved digestive health:**
   Fiber adds bulk to your stool and helps regulate bowel movements, preventing constipation and promoting regularity. It can also help alleviate symptoms of conditions like irritable bowel syndrome (IBS) and diverticulosis.

2. **Weight management:**
   High-fiber foods are generally more filling and can help you feel satisfied for longer periods, which can aid in weight management by reducing overall calorie intake. Fiber-rich foods also tend to be lower in calories and higher in nutrients than processed foods.

3. **Blood sugar control:**
Soluble fiber, found in foods like oats, legumes, and fruits, can help slow down the absorption of sugar into the bloodstream, preventing spikes in blood sugar levels. This can be beneficial for individuals with diabetes or those at risk of developing it.

4. **Heart health:**
A high-fiber diet has been associated with a reduced risk of heart disease. Soluble fiber helps lower LDL (bad) cholesterol levels by binding to cholesterol and removing it from the body. It can also help regulate blood pressure and reduce inflammation.

5. **Weight maintenance:**
High-fiber foods are often less energy-dense and can help you feel full without consuming excessive calories. This can be beneficial for maintaining a healthy weight or achieving weight loss goals.

6. **Reduced risk of certain cancers:**
Adequate fiber intake, particularly from whole grains, fruits, and vegetables, has been linked to a lower risk of colorectal cancer. Fiber helps promote healthy digestion and may help remove potential carcinogens from the colon.

7. **Improved gut health:**
   Fiber acts as a prebiotic, providing nourishment for beneficial gut bacteria. This can help support a healthy gut microbiome, which is essential for optimal digestion, nutrient absorption, and overall immune function.

8. **Lower risk of chronic diseases:**
   A high-fiber diet has been associated with a reduced risk of various chronic diseases, including type 2 diabetes, stroke, and certain types of cancer. The combination of fiber's effects on blood sugar control, cholesterol levels, and weight management contributes to these benefits.

It's important to note that increasing fiber intake should be done gradually to avoid digestive discomfort. Aim for a variety of fiber sources, including fruits, vegetables, whole grains, legumes, nuts, and seeds, to obtain the full range of benefits that dietary fiber offers.

5.2 HIGH-FIBER FOODS TO INCLUDE IN YOUR DIET

Including high-fiber foods in your diet is a great way to increase your fiber intake. Here are some examples of high-fiber foods that you can include:

1. **WHOLE GRAINS:**
   Whole wheat, oats, brown rice, quinoa, and barley are excellent sources of dietary fiber. Choose whole grain bread, pasta, and cereals over refined grains to maximize your fiber intake.

2. **FRUITS:**
   Many fruits are high in fiber. Examples include raspberries, blackberries, pears, apples, bananas, oranges, and strawberries. Aim to eat the skin of fruits whenever possible, as it often contains additional fiber.

3. **VEGETABLES**:
   Vegetables are generally high in fiber. Some fiber-rich options include broccoli, Brussels sprouts, carrots, spinach, kale, artichokes, and sweet potatoes. Incorporate a variety of vegetables into your meals and snacks to increase your fiber intake.

4. **LEGUMES:**
   Beans, lentils, chickpeas, and other legumes are rich sources of fiber. They are also high in protein and can be used in soups, stews, salads, or as a side dish.

5. **NUTS AND SEEDS:**
Almonds, walnuts, chia seeds, palm kernel, flaxseeds, and sunflower seeds are all high in fiber. Enjoy them as a snack, sprinkle them on salads or yogurt, or use them in baking and cooking.

6. **AVOCADO:**
Avocado is a unique fruit that is high in fiber, healthy fats, and various nutrients. Add slices of avocado to sandwiches, salads, or use it as a spread instead of butter or mayonnaise.

7. **BERRIES:**
Berries like raspberries, blackberries, and blueberries are not only delicious but also high in fiber. Enjoy them fresh, frozen, or add them to smoothies, yogurt, or oatmeal.

8. **BRAN:**
Wheat bran, oat bran, and rice bran are concentrated sources of fiber. You can sprinkle them on cereal, yogurt, or use them in baking recipes to increase your fiber intake.

Remember to increase your fiber intake gradually and drink plenty of water to help prevent digestive discomfort. Aim to include a variety of high-fiber foods in your diet to ensure you're getting a range of nutrients along with the fiber.

5.3 CREATIVE WAYS TO INCREASE FIBER INTAKE

Increasing fiber intake can be fun and creative! Here are some innovative ways to incorporate more fiber into your diet:

1. **VEGGIE NOODLES:**
   Instead of traditional pasta, try making noodles from vegetables like zucchini, sweet potatoes, or carrots using a spiralizer. These veggie noodles are high in fiber and can be used as a base for your favorite pasta dishes.

2. **FIBER-RICH SMOOTHIES:**
   Blend fiber-rich fruits like berries, bananas, and mangoes with leafy greens like spinach or kale. You can also add a tablespoon of chia seeds or ground flaxseeds for an extra fiber boost.

3. **FIBER-PACKED TOPPINGS:**
   Sprinkle fiber-rich toppings like chia seeds, ground flaxseeds, or hemp seeds on your yogurt, oatmeal, or salads. These small additions can significantly increase your fiber intake.

 ANTI-CANCER FOODS | By Pst. Engr. Emeka Unaegbu

4. **BEAN-BASED DESSERTS:**
Experiment with desserts made from beans, such as black bean brownies or chickpea cookie dough. These recipes are not only delicious but also provide a good amount of fiber.

5. **FIBER-RICH SNACKS:**
Opt for high-fiber snacks like air-popped popcorn, roasted chickpeas, or homemade granola bars packed with nuts, seeds, and dried fruits.

6. **FIBER-FILLED WRAPS AND SANDWICHES**:
Use whole grain or whole wheat wraps or bread for your sandwiches. Fill them with fiber-rich ingredients like avocado, leafy greens, sprouts, and lean proteins for a satisfying and high-fiber meal.

7. **FIBER-PACKED SALADS:**
Load your salads with a variety of vegetables, legumes, nuts, and seeds. Add ingredients like roasted sweet potatoes, quinoa, or edamame to boost the fiber content.

8. **FIBER-RICH BREAKFAST BOWLS**:
Start your day with a fiber-filled breakfast bowl. Combine fiber-rich ingredients like oats, chia seeds,

berries, almonds, and Greek yogurt for a nutritious and filling meal.

9. **HIGH-FIBER SOUPS:**
Prepare homemade soups using fiber-rich ingredients like lentils, beans, vegetables, and whole grains. These hearty soups are not only delicious but also provide a good amount of fiber.

10. **FIBER-ADDED BAKING:**
Add fiber-rich ingredients like bran, ground flaxseeds, or whole wheat flour to your baking recipes. This can be done in muffins, bread, pancakes, or cookies.

Remember to gradually increase your fiber intake and drink plenty of water to help with digestion. These creative and innovative ways can make increasing fiber intake enjoyable and delicious.

CHAPTER SIX

AVOIDING CARCINOGENS AND HARMFUL SUBSTANCES IN YOUR DIET

6.1 IDENTIFYING CARCINOGENS IN FOODS AND BEVERAGES

There are several carcinogens and harmful substances that can be present in our diet. Here are a few examples:

1. **PROCESSED MEATS:**
Processed meats like bacon, sausages, hot dogs, and deli meats are classified as Group 1 carcinogens by the International Agency for Research on Cancer (IARC). These meats undergo processes like curing, smoking, or adding preservatives, which can lead to the formation of harmful substances like nitrosamines.

2. **ACRYLAMIDE:**
Acrylamide is a chemical compound that forms naturally in starchy foods when they are cooked at high temperatures, such as during frying, baking, or roasting. It is found in foods like French fries, potato

chips, and roasted coffee. Acrylamide has been classified as a probable human carcinogen.

3. **POLYCYCLIC AROMATIC HYDROCARBONS (PAHS):**

PAHs are a group of chemicals that can be formed when meat, poultry, or fish is cooked at high temperatures, such as grilling or barbecuing. PAHs have been linked to an increased risk of cancer, particularly when meat is charred or exposed to high levels of smoke.

4. **HETEROCYCLIC AMINES (HCAS) AND POLYCYCLIC AROMATIC HYDROCARBONS (PAHS):**

HCAs and PAHs are formed when meat, poultry, or fish is cooked at high temperatures, such as grilling, frying, or broiling. These compounds have been associated with an increased risk of certain cancers, including colorectal, pancreatic, and prostate cancer.

5. **TRANS FATS:**

Tran's fats are artificially created fats that are commonly found in processed and fried foods, baked goods, and margarine. Tran's fats have been linked to an increased risk of heart disease and are considered harmful to overall health.

6. **ADDED SUGARS:**
Consuming excessive amounts of added sugars, such as those found in sugary drinks, desserts, candies, and processed foods, can contribute to weight gain, obesity, and an increased risk of chronic diseases like type 2 diabetes and certain types of cancer.

It's important to note that the risk associated with these substances may depend on the frequency and quantity consumed. To reduce exposure to harmful substances, it is recommended to focus on a balanced diet that includes a variety of whole, unprocessed foods and to limit the consumption of processed meats, fried foods, and foods high in added sugars. Additionally, cooking methods that involve lower temperatures and shorter cooking times can help reduce the formation of harmful compounds.

6.2 TIPS FOR REDUCING EXPOSURE TO HARMFUL SUBSTANCES

Reducing exposure to harmful substances in your diet is important for maintaining good health. Here are some tips to help you minimize your exposure:

1. **CHOOSE WHOLE, UNPROCESSED FOODS:**
Opt for whole foods like fruits, vegetables, whole grains, lean proteins, and legumes. These foods are generally lower in harmful substances compared to processed and packaged foods.

2. **LIMIT PROCESSED MEATS:**
Processed meats like bacon, sausages, and deli meats have been linked to increased health risks. Minimize your consumption of these meats and choose lean, unprocessed alternatives like poultry, fish, or plant-based proteins.

3. **PRACTICE HEALTHY COOKING METHODS**:
Avoid high-temperature cooking methods like frying, grilling, or barbecuing, which can lead to the formation of harmful compounds. Instead, opt for steaming, boiling, baking, or sautéing at lower temperatures.

4. **REDUCE ACRYLAMIDE FORMATION:**
To minimize acrylamide formation in foods, avoid overcooking or burning starchy foods like potatoes, bread, and cereals. Opt for lighter cooking methods like baking or boiling instead of deep frying or high-temperature cooking.

5. **LIMIT EXPOSURE TO FOOD ADDITIVES:**
Read food labels and avoid foods that contain artificial additives, preservatives, and colorings. Choose foods with minimal ingredients and opt for natural alternatives whenever possible.

6. **MINIMIZE CONSUMPTION OF SUGARY FOODS AND DRINKS:**
Limit your intake of sugary drinks, desserts, candies, and processed foods high in added sugars. Instead, satisfy your sweet tooth with naturally sweet foods like fruits or homemade treats with reduced sugar.

7. **CHOOSE ORGANIC PRODUCE:**
Consider opting for organic produce, which is grown without the use of synthetic pesticides, herbicides, and fertilizers. This can help reduce exposure to potentially harmful chemicals.

8. **STAY HYDRATED:**
Drinking plenty of water can help flush out toxins from your body and support overall health. Aim to drink an adequate amount of water throughout the day.

9. **PRACTICE PORTION CONTROL:**
Overconsumption of any food, even healthy ones, can have negative effects on your health. Practice portion control to ensure a balanced diet and avoid excessive exposure to harmful substances.

10. **MAINTAIN A BALANCED DIET:**
Focus on a balanced diet that includes a variety of nutrient-rich foods. This can help ensure you're getting a range of beneficial nutrients while minimizing exposure to harmful substances.

Remember, it's important to make sustainable changes to your eating habits over time. Incorporate these tips gradually into your lifestyle to reduce exposure to harmful substances and promote overall health.

6.3 SAFE COOKING AND FOOD PREPARATION PRACTICES

Practicing safe cooking and food preparation practices is essential to prevent foodborne illnesses and ensure the safety of the food you consume. Here are some tips to follow:

1. **CLEANLINESS:**
Wash your hands thoroughly with soap and warm water for at least 20 seconds before handling food.

Clean and sanitize kitchen surfaces, utensils, and cutting boards regularly to avoid cross-contamination.

2. **SEPARATION:**
Keep raw meats, poultry, seafood, and eggs separate from other foods to prevent the spread of bacteria. Use separate cutting boards and utensils for raw and cooked foods.

3. **PROPER STORAGE:**
Store perishable foods, such as meat, dairy products, and leftovers, in the refrigerator at or below 40°F (4°C) to slow down bacterial growth. Use airtight containers or wraps to prevent cross-contamination and maintain food quality.

4. **THOROUGH COOKING:**
Cook foods to the appropriate internal temperature to kill harmful bacteria. Use a food thermometer to ensure that meat, poultry, fish, and eggs are cooked to the recommended safe temperatures.

5. **AVOID CROSS-CONTAMINATION:**
Prevent cross-contamination by keeping raw and cooked foods separate. Don't use the same utensils, cutting boards, or plates for raw and cooked foods without proper cleaning in between.

6. **PROPER THAWING:**
Thaw frozen foods in the refrigerator, under cold running water, or in the microwave using the defrost setting. Avoid thawing foods at room temperature, as it can promote bacterial growth.

7. **SAFE LEFTOVERS:**
Refrigerate or freeze leftovers promptly after cooking. Use cooked leftovers within 3-4 days, and reheat them to an internal temperature of 165°F (74°C) before consuming.

8. **AVOIDING EXPIRED OR SPOILED FOOD**:
Check expiration dates on food packages and discard any expired or spoiled items. Trust your senses – if a food looks, smells, or tastes off, it's better to be safe and discard it.

9. **SAFE HANDLING OF PRODUCE:**
Wash fresh fruits and vegetables thoroughly under running water before consuming or preparing them. Use a produce brush to scrub firm produce like potatoes or cucumbers.

10. **SAFE REHEATING:**
When reheating food, make sure it reaches a temperature of 165°F (74°C) throughout to kill any bacteria that may have grown during storage.

By following these safe cooking and food preparation practices, you can significantly reduce the risk of foodborne illnesses and ensure the safety of the food you consume.

CHAPTER SEVEN

THE IMPORTANCE OF HYDRATION IN CANCER PREVENTION

Hydration plays a crucial role in overall health, including cancer prevention. While there isn't direct evidence that links hydration to cancer prevention, maintaining proper hydration levels is essential for supporting the body's overall functions and reducing certain cancer risk factors. Here's how hydration can contribute to cancer prevention:

1. **PROMOTES OVERALL HEALTH:**
   Staying properly hydrated is important for maintaining overall health and well-being. It supports various bodily functions, including digestion, circulation, and detoxification. When your body is functioning optimally, it can better defend against cancerous cells and maintain a healthy immune system.

2. **SUPPORTS DETOXIFICATION:**
   Adequate hydration helps flush toxins and waste products from the body. Proper hydration supports the kidneys' ability to filter and eliminate waste, reducing the burden on other detoxification organs, such as the liver. This can help reduce the risk of

exposure to harmful substances that may contribute to cancer development.

3. **AIDS IN DIGESTION AND BOWEL REGULARITY**:
Staying hydrated helps maintain proper digestion and bowel regularity. Sufficient water intake can prevent constipation and promote the elimination of waste products from the body. This reduces the duration of exposure of the digestive system to potentially harmful substances, which may be linked to certain types of cancer, such as colorectal cancer.

4. **SUPPORTS A HEALTHY WEIGHT:**
Proper hydration can contribute to maintaining a healthy weight, which is an important factor in cancer prevention. Drinking water before meals can help reduce calorie intake and promote a feeling of fullness, potentially leading to weight management or weight loss. Obesity is associated with an increased risk of several types of cancer.

5. **MAINTAINS HEALTHY CELLS AND TISSUES:**
Hydration is important for maintaining the health and integrity of cells and tissues throughout the body. Sufficient water intake helps transport nutrients to cells, supports proper cell function, and aids in the removal of metabolic waste products.

Healthy cells and tissues are less prone to mutations and abnormalities that can lead to cancer development.

While hydration is an important aspect of a healthy lifestyle, it is just one factor among many that contribute to cancer prevention. It is crucial to adopt a comprehensive approach to reduce cancer risks, including maintaining a balanced diet, engaging in regular physical activity, avoiding tobacco and excessive alcohol consumption, and getting regular screenings as recommended by healthcare professionals.

7.2 TIPS FOR STAYING HYDRATED AND CHOOSING HEALTHY BEVERAGES

Staying hydrated is essential for overall health and well-being. Here are some tips to help you stay hydrated and choose healthy beverages:

1. **DRINK WATER REGULARLY:**
   Water is the best choice for staying hydrated. Keep a water bottle with you throughout the day and sip on it regularly. Aim to drink at least 8 cups (64 ounces) of water per day, or more if you are physically active or in hot weather.

2. **INFUSE WATER WITH FLAVOR:**
   If you find plain water boring, infuse it with natural flavors like slices of citrus fruits, berries, or herbs like mint or basil. This can add a refreshing taste without any added sugars or artificial ingredients.

3. **LIMIT SUGARY DRINKS:**
   Sugary drinks like soda, fruit juices, energy drinks, and sweetened teas can be high in calories and added sugars. Limit your consumption of these beverages as they can contribute to weight gain and other health issues. Instead, choose healthier alternatives.

4. **CHOOSE UNSWEETENED HERBAL TEAS:**
   Herbal teas can be a hydrating and flavorful option. Opt for unsweetened varieties and experiment with different flavors like chamomile, green tea, or hibiscus.

5. **INCLUDE LOW-FAT OR SKIM MILK:**
   Milk is not only a good source of hydration but also provides essential nutrients like calcium and protein. Choose low-fat or skim milk to keep the calorie and fat content in check.

6. **CONSUME NATURAL FRUIT JUICES IN MODERATION**:
If you enjoy fruit juices, choose 100% natural juices without added sugars or artificial additives. However, it's important to consume them in moderation due to their natural sugar content.

7. **BE CAUTIOUS WITH SPORTS DRINKS**:
Sports drinks are designed to replenish electrolytes and provide energy during intense physical activity or prolonged exercise. If you engage in such activities, sports drinks can be beneficial. However, for everyday hydration needs, water is usually sufficient.

8. **LIMIT CAFFEINATED BEVERAGES**:
Caffeinated beverages like coffee, tea, and some soft drinks can have a diuretic effect, meaning they may increase urine production and potentially contribute to dehydration. While moderate consumption is generally fine, it's best to balance caffeinated beverages with adequate water intake.

9. **MONITOR ALCOHOL INTAKE:**
Alcohol can dehydrate the body, so it's important to consume alcoholic beverages in moderation. Drink water alongside alcoholic beverages and pace yourself to minimize the dehydrating effects.

10. **MONITOR YOUR URINE COLOR:**
A simple way to check your hydration status is by monitoring the color of your urine. Pale yellow or clear urine generally indicates good hydration, while darker urine may indicate dehydration.

Remember, individual hydration needs may vary depending on factors like activity level, climate, and overall health. Listen to your body's thirst cues and make a conscious effort to stay hydrated throughout the day.

CHAPTER EIGHT

CREATING A CANCER-PREVENTIVE MEAL PLAN

8.1 PLANNING YOUR MEALS FOR OPTIMAL CANCER PREVENTION

Planning your meals with a focus on cancer prevention involves incorporating a variety of nutrient-rich foods that are known to have cancer-fighting properties. Here are some tips to help you plan meals for optimal cancer prevention:

1. **INCLUDE A VARIETY OF FRUITS AND VEGETABLES:**
   Aim to fill half of your plate with a colorful assortment of fruits and vegetables. These plant-based foods are rich in vitamins, minerals, antioxidants, and fiber, which have been linked to a reduced risk of various cancers. Include a mix of leafy greens, cruciferous vegetables (such as broccoli, cauliflower, and Brussels sprouts), berries, citrus fruits, and other colorful produce.

2. **CHOOSE WHOLE GRAINS:**
   Opt for whole grains like brown rice, quinoa, whole wheat bread, and oats instead of refined grains. Whole grains are high in fiber, vitamins, minerals,

and antioxidants, which can help reduce the risk of certain cancers. They also provide sustained energy and promote overall health.

3. **INCLUDE LEAN PROTEINS:**
Incorporate lean sources of protein like poultry, fish, beans, lentils, tofu, and Greek yogurt. These protein sources are lower in saturated fats compared to red and processed meats, which have been associated with an increased risk of certain cancers. Plant-based proteins also provide additional phytochemicals and fiber that can support cancer prevention.

4. **LIMIT RED AND PROCESSED MEATS:**
Red meats like beef, pork, and lamb, as well as processed meats like bacon, sausages, and deli meats, have been linked to an increased risk of certain cancers. Limit your consumption of these meats and choose leaner alternatives like poultry or fish. If you do consume red or processed meats, opt for smaller portions and less frequent consumption.

5. **INCLUDE HEALTHY FATS:**
Incorporate sources of healthy fats into your meals, such as avocados, nuts, seeds, and olive oil. These fats provide essential nutrients and can help reduce

inflammation in the body, which is a risk factor for cancer development. However, moderation is key, as fats are high in calories, so be mindful of portion sizes.

6. **MINIMIZE PROCESSED AND PACKAGED FOODS:**
Processed and packaged foods often contain high levels of added sugars, unhealthy fats, and artificial additives. These can contribute to weight gain and increase the risk of certain cancers. Focus on whole, unprocessed foods and limit your intake of processed snacks, sugary drinks, and pre-packaged meals.

7. **SPICE IT UP WITH HERBS AND SPICES**:
Many herbs and spices have potent antioxidant and anti-inflammatory properties that can support cancer prevention. Include herbs and spices like turmeric, ginger, garlic, cinnamon, oregano, and rosemary in your meals to add flavor and potential health benefits.

8. **STAY HYDRATED:**
Adequate hydration is important for overall health, including cancer prevention. Drink plenty of water throughout the day and limit the consumption of sugary drinks.

9. **PRACTICE PORTION CONTROL:**
   Be mindful of portion sizes to maintain a healthy weight and balance your nutrient intake. Overeating can lead to weight gain, which is a risk factor for certain cancers.

10. **LIMIT ALCOHOL CONSUMPTION**:
   Excessive alcohol consumption has been linked to an increased risk of several cancers. If you choose to drink alcohol, do so in moderation. The American Cancer Society recommends limiting alcohol intake to no more than one drink per day for women and two drinks per day for men.

Remember, a healthy and balanced diet is just one aspect of cancer prevention. It's also important to maintain a physically active lifestyle, avoid tobacco and excessive alcohol consumption, protect yourself from the sun, and get regular screenings as recommended by healthcare professionals.

8.2 SAMPLE MEAL PLAN FOR CANCER-PREVENTION DIET

Here's a sample meal plan that incorporates cancer-fighting foods and follows a balanced, nutrient-rich approach:

ANTI-CANCER FOODS | By Pst. Engr. Emeka Unaegbu

BREAKFAST:

- Overnight oats made with rolled oats, almond milk, chia seeds, and topped with berries and a sprinkle of ground flaxseeds.
- A side of sliced avocado and a cup of green tea.

SNACK:

- A handful of mixed nuts (such as almonds, walnuts, and cashews).
- A piece of fresh fruit, like an apple or a handful of grapes.

LUNCH:

- Mixed green salad with a variety of colorful vegetables (such as spinach, kale, cherry tomatoes, cucumber, and bell peppers).
- Grilled chicken breast or chickpeas for plant-based protein.
- Tossed with a homemade vinaigrette made with olive oil, lemon juice, Dijon mustard, and herbs.
- A side of whole grain bread or quinoa.

SNACK:

- Carrot sticks and hummus dip.
- A cup of herbal tea.

DINNER:

- Baked salmon or tofu marinated in a mixture of lemon juice, garlic, and herbs.
- Steamed broccoli and cauliflower.
- Quinoa or brown rice as a side dish.

SNACK:

- Greek yogurt topped with fresh berries and a sprinkle of granola.

Remember to adjust portion sizes based on your individual needs and consult with a healthcare professional or registered dietitian for personalized advice. This sample meal plan provides a general idea of how to incorporate cancer-preventive foods into your diet, but it's important to maintain a varied and balanced eating pattern.

8.3 ADJUSTING THE MEAL PLAN TO INDIVIDUAL DIETARY NEEDS

Certainly! Here's an adjusted version of the sample meal plan to accommodate different dietary needs:

BREAKFAST:

- Overnight oats made with gluten-free oats or a gluten-free alternative like quinoa flakes, almond

milk, chia seeds, and topped with berries and a sprinkle of ground flaxseeds.
- A side of sliced avocado and a cup of herbal tea.

SNACK:
- A handful of mixed seeds (such as pumpkin seeds, sunflower seeds, and hemp seeds).
- A piece of fresh fruit, like a pear or a handful of blueberries.

LUNCH:
- Mixed green salad with a variety of colorful vegetables (such as spinach, arugula, cherry tomatoes, cucumber, and bell peppers).
- Grilled tofu or tempeh for plant-based protein.
- Tossed with a homemade dressing made with olive oil, apple cider vinegar, Dijon mustard, and herbs.
- A side of gluten-free bread or quinoa.

SNACK:
- Rice cakes or gluten-free crackers with almond butter or hummus.
- A cup of herbal tea or infused water.

DINNER:

- Baked chicken breast or fish (choose a variety that suits your dietary needs) marinated in a mixture of lemon juice, garlic, and herbs.
- Steamed or roasted vegetables like asparagus, zucchini, and carrots.
- Quinoa, brown rice, or a gluten-free grain as a side dish.

SNACK:

- Dairy-free yogurt (such as coconut or almond milk-based) topped with fresh berries and a sprinkle of gluten-free granola.

Remember to adjust portion sizes and ingredients based on your specific dietary needs and preferences. It's always a good idea to consult with a healthcare professional or registered dietitian for personalized guidance and to ensure that your meal plan meets your individual requirements.

CHAPTER NINE

LIFESTYLE FACTORS TO SUPPORT CANCER PREVENTION

9.1 REGULAR PHYSICAL ACTIVITY AND CANCER PREVENTION

Regular physical activity plays a crucial role in cancer prevention. Here's how it can help reduce the risk of developing certain types of cancer:

1. **WEIGHT MANAGEMENT:**
   Engaging in regular physical activity can help maintain a healthy weight or promote weight loss. Being overweight or obese is a known risk factor for several types of cancer, including breast, colorectal, endometrial, kidney, and pancreatic cancer. By maintaining a healthy weight, you can reduce the risk of developing these cancers.

2. **HORMONE REGULATION:**
   Physical activity can help regulate hormone levels in the body. High levels of certain hormones, such as estrogen, have been linked to an increased risk of breast and endometrial cancer. Regular exercise can help lower estrogen levels and reduce the risk of these hormone-related cancers.

3. **IMPROVED IMMUNE FUNCTION:**
Regular physical activity can enhance the immune system's function, making it more effective in fighting off cancer cells and preventing the development of tumors.

4. **REDUCED INFLAMMATION:**
Chronic inflammation in the body is associated with an increased risk of cancer. Exercise helps reduce inflammation and promotes a healthier inflammatory response, which can lower the risk of cancer development.

5. **IMPROVED DIGESTION:**
Physical activity can help regulate digestion and promote regular bowel movements. This can reduce the risk of colorectal cancer, as prolonged exposure to waste products in the colon can increase the likelihood of cancerous changes.

6. **ENHANCED INSULIN SENSITIVITY:**
Regular exercise improves insulin sensitivity, reducing the risk of insulin resistance and type 2 diabetes. High insulin levels have been linked to an increased risk of several types of cancer, including breast, colorectal, and pancreatic cancer.

7. **STRESS REDUCTION:**
Physical activity is known to reduce stress levels and improve mental well-being. Chronic stress can weaken the immune system and increase the risk of cancer. Engaging in regular exercise can help manage stress and promote overall health.

To incorporate physical activity into your routine for cancer prevention, aim for at least 150 minutes of moderate-intensity aerobic activity or 75 minutes of vigorous-intensity aerobic activity per week. Additionally, include strength training exercises at least twice a week to build and maintain muscle mass.

Remember to choose activities that you enjoy, as this will increase the likelihood of sticking with a regular exercise routine. Consult with a healthcare professional before starting any new exercise program, especially if you have underlying health conditions or concerns.

9.2 MANAGING STRESS AND IT'S IMPACT ON CANCER RISKS

Managing stress is important not only for your overall well-being but also for reducing the risk of cancer. Chronic stress can have negative effects on your immune system, hormone levels, and inflammation levels, all of which can contribute to an increased risk of cancer. Here are some strategies to help you manage stress and minimize its impact on cancer risks:

1. **REGULAR EXERCISE:**
   Engaging in physical activity can help reduce stress levels by releasing endorphins, improving mood, and promoting relaxation. Aim for at least 150 minutes of moderate-intensity aerobic activity or 75 minutes of vigorous-intensity aerobic activity per week, along with strength training exercises.

2. **PRACTICE RELAXATION TECHNIQUES:**
   Incorporate relaxation techniques into your daily routine, such as deep breathing exercises, meditation, yoga, or tai chi. These practices can help calm the mind, reduce stress, and promote a sense of well-being.

3. **PRIORITIZE SELF-CARE:**
   Take time for self-care activities that you enjoy, such as reading, taking baths, listening to music, or engaging in hobbies. These activities can help you relax and unwind, reducing stress levels.

4. **MAINTAIN A BALANCED LIFESTYLE:**
   Strive for a balanced lifestyle by setting boundaries, prioritizing your needs, and managing your time

effectively. This can help reduce feelings of overwhelm and stress.

5. **SEEK SOCIAL SUPPORT:**
Reach out to friends, family, or support groups for emotional support. Sharing your feelings and experiences with others can help alleviate stress and provide a sense of connection and understanding.

6. **PRACTICE STRESS-REDUCING TECHNIQUES:**
Find stress-reducing techniques that work for you, such as journaling, practicing gratitude, engaging in creative outlets, or engaging in activities that bring you joy.

7. **GET ENOUGH SLEEP:**
Prioritize getting enough quality sleep each night. Lack of sleep can contribute to increased stress levels and negatively impact your overall health. Aim for 7-9 hours of uninterrupted sleep per night.

8. **LIMIT EXPOSURE TO STRESSORS:**
Identify and limit exposure to stressors in your life, whether they be certain people, situations, or environments. If possible, make changes to reduce or eliminate these stressors.

 ANTI-CANCER FOODS | By Pst. Engr. Emeka Unaegbu

9. **SEEK PROFESSIONAL HELP IF NEEDED:**
If you find that stress is overwhelming and impacting your daily life, consider seeking professional help from a therapist or counselor who can provide guidance and support.

Remember, managing stress is a lifelong practice, and what works for one person may not work for another. It's important to find stress management techniques that resonate with you and incorporate them into your daily routine. By effectively managing stress, you can reduce its impact on your overall health and lower the risk of cancer.

9.3 OTHER HEALTHY LIFESTYLE HABITS FOR CANCER PREVENTION

In addition to regular physical activity and stress management, there are several other healthy lifestyle habits that can help reduce the risk of cancer. Here are some key recommendations:

1. **HEALTHY DIET:**
Follow a balanced, nutrient-rich diet that includes plenty of fruits, vegetables, whole grains, lean proteins, and healthy fats. Limit processed foods, sugary drinks, and red and processed meats. Aim

for a variety of colors on your plate to ensure you're getting a wide range of cancer-fighting nutrients.

2. **MAINTAIN A HEALTHY WEIGHT:**
Strive to maintain a healthy weight through a combination of regular physical activity and a balanced diet. Excess body weight, especially around the waist, is linked to an increased risk of several types of cancer.

3. **LIMIT ALCOHOL CONSUMPTION:**
If you choose to drink alcohol, do so in moderation. For women, this means up to one drink per day, and for men, up to two drinks per day. Excessive alcohol consumption is associated with an increased risk of various cancers, including breast, liver, colorectal, and mouth cancers.

4. **QUIT SMOKING:**
If you smoke, quitting is the best thing you can do for your health. Smoking is a leading cause of various types of cancer, including lung, mouth, throat, esophageal, and pancreatic cancer. Seek support from healthcare professionals or smoking cessation programs to help you quit.

5. **PROTECT YOURSELF FROM THE SUN:**
Limit exposure to the sun's harmful ultraviolet (UV) rays, especially between 10 a.m. and 4 p.m. when the sun is strongest. Use sunscreen with a high SPF, wear protective clothing, and seek shade whenever possible. Avoid tanning beds and sunlamps, as they also emit harmful UV radiation.

6. **GET VACCINATED:**
Certain infections can increase the risk of developing cancer. Protect yourself by getting vaccinated against hepatitis B, which can cause liver cancer, and human papillomavirus (HPV), which can lead to cervical, anal, and other types of cancer.

7. **PRACTICE SAFE SEX:**
Engage in safe sexual practices to reduce the risk of sexually transmitted infections, such as HPV, which can increase the risk of certain cancers.

8. **STAY UP TO DATE WITH CANCER SCREENINGS**:
Regular screenings can help detect cancer at early stages when it's most treatable. Follow recommended guidelines for screenings, such as mammograms, Pap tests, colonoscopies, and prostate exams, based on your age, gender, and family history.

9. **LIMIT EXPOSURE TO ENVIRONMENTAL TOXINS**:
Minimize exposure to environmental toxins, such as asbestos, radon, and certain chemicals. Take necessary precautions at work or in your living environment to reduce exposure to these substances.

Remember, no lifestyle change can guarantee the prevention of cancer, but adopting these healthy habits can significantly reduce your risk. It's essential to consult with healthcare professionals for personalized advice and to follow recommended guidelines for cancer screenings based on your individual circumstances.

CHAPTER TEN

CONCLUSION

Incorporating a healthy diet into your lifestyle is an important aspect of cancer prevention. While no specific food or diet can completely eliminate the risk of cancer, research suggests that certain dietary choices can help reduce the likelihood of developing the disease. Emphasize on plant-based foods such as Fruits, vegetables, whole grains, legumes, and nuts are rich in vitamins, minerals, antioxidants, and fiber, which have been associated with a lower risk of various types of cancer. Aim to fill at least half of your plate with a variety of colorful plant-based foods.

Choose lean proteins by opting for lean sources of protein, such as poultry, fish, beans, lentils, and tofu. Limit red and processed meats, as they have been linked to an increased risk of colorectal and other cancers.

Limit processed and sugary foods, highly processed foods, sugary snacks, and beverages have been associated with an increased risk of obesity and certain types of cancer. Minimize your intake of these foods and focus on whole, unprocessed options.

Be mindful of portion sizes, even healthy foods should be consumed in moderation. Pay attention to portion sizes to avoid overeating and maintain a healthy weight.

Stay hydrated by drinking plenty of water throughout the day to stay properly hydrated. Limit sugary drinks and opt for water, herbal tea, or infused water instead.

Also practice mindful eating, by slowing down and paying attention to your body's hunger and fullness cues. Mindful eating can help prevent overeating and promote a healthier relationship with food.

Limit alcohol consumption, since excessive alcohol consumption has been linked to an increased risk of various cancers. If you choose to drink, do so in moderation or consider avoiding alcohol altogether.

Consult professional for specific dietary concerns or health conditions, consult with a registered dietitian or healthcare professional who can provide personalized recommendations and guidance.

Finally remember, a healthy diet is just one component of a comprehensive approach to cancer prevention. It's important to combine it with other lifestyle factors such as regular physical activity, stress management, not smoking, and following recommended screenings and vaccinations. By adopting a holistic approach, you can significantly reduce your risk of developing cancer and improve your overall well-being. It is rewarding to be in good health, and once you are practicing what have been elucidated in this book, chances are that you will be in good health and vitality to achieve your life dreams. Starting early in life in practicing these health tips is key to good health and longevity devoid of cancer and other related life threatening illnesses. A stitch in time saves nine.

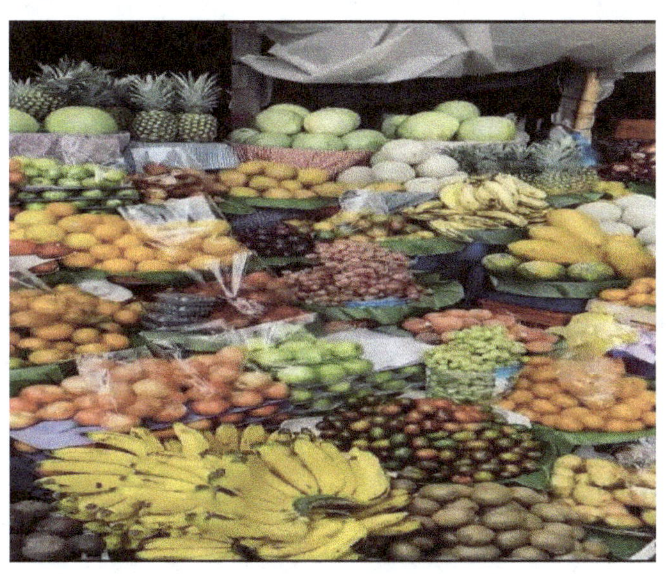

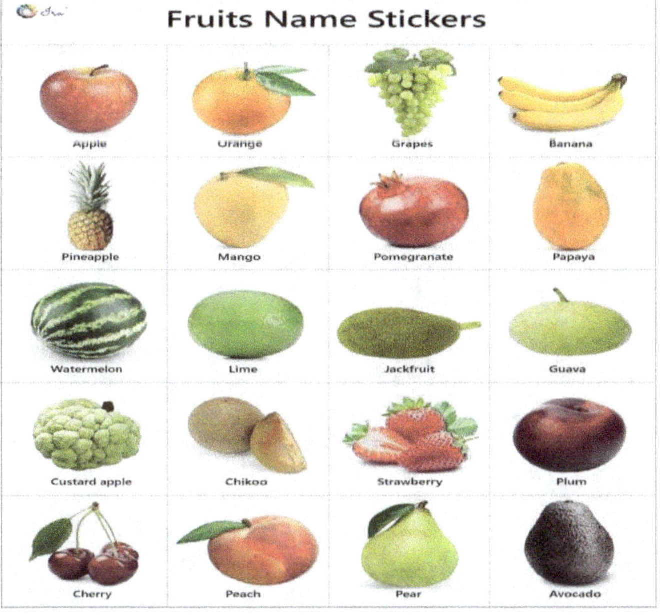

ANTI-CANCER FOODS | By Pst. Engr. Emeka Unaegbu